In My Dreams

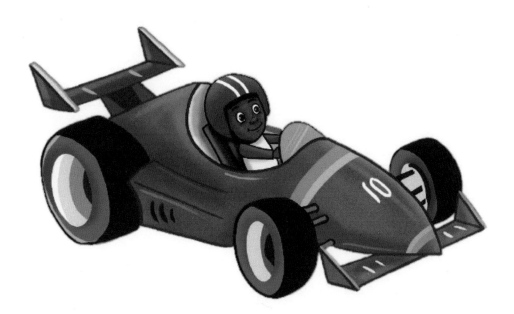

Michelle Marshall

Published by

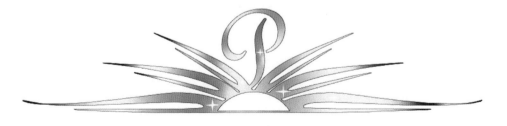

Peaches

Publications

With love

Erran

Keep dreaming

Michelle Clar

Published in London by Peaches Publications LTD, 2022.

www.peachespublications.co.uk

British Library Cataloguing in Publication Data: A catalogue record for this book is available from the British Library.

ISBN: 9781739793296

Book cover design: Peaches Publications and Michelle Marshall.

Editor: Winsome Duncan.

Typesetter: Winsome Duncan.

Proofreader: Virginia Rounding.

Dedication

This book is inspired by all children and young people living
with a disability of any kind.

For your courage I dedicate this book to you.

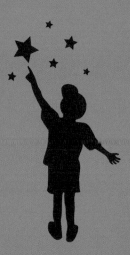

Acknowledgements

I was inspired to write this book because of some amazing opportunities I have had to work with incredible children and young people with various challenges.

It was a humbling experience observing them as they encountered and conquered their environment.

I am motivated by the children and young people's strength, determination, courage and resilience.

Children are brave and explorative individuals, who inspired me to adopt a similar attitude, which has greatly helped me in my life endeavours.

This book is to inspire you past your limitations and encourage you that, no matter what your race, ethnicity, age or gender, you are capable of amazing things and deserve happiness.

I give a special thanks to my family, who have continuously supported me throughout the writing process. I appreciate everything they have done for me to make this book possible.

I am eternally grateful for their contribution to my life.

I would also like to give special thanks to Winsome Duncan, CEO of Peaches Publications, for making this book a reality.

The support during a very turbulent pandemic has given way for creativity to finally come alive.

In loving memory of Ronald Foster Lynch

13.05.1937- 13.06.2022

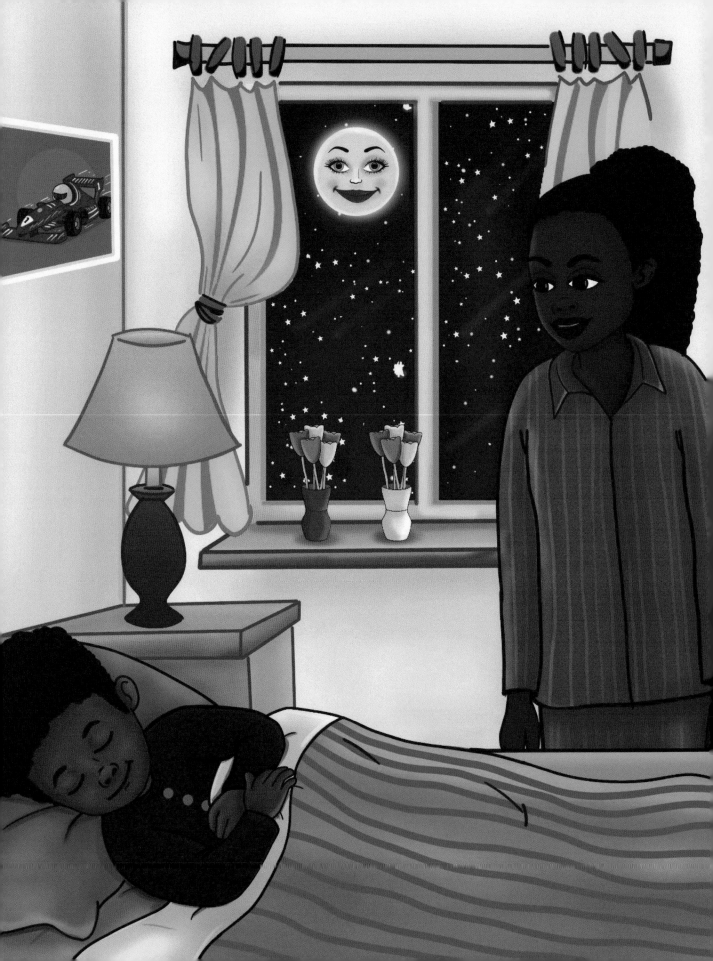

As I count the stars at night, my mother comes in
and says "sleep tight".
She tucks me in and kisses my chin.
This is where my journey begins!

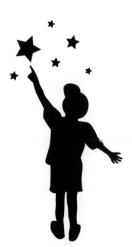

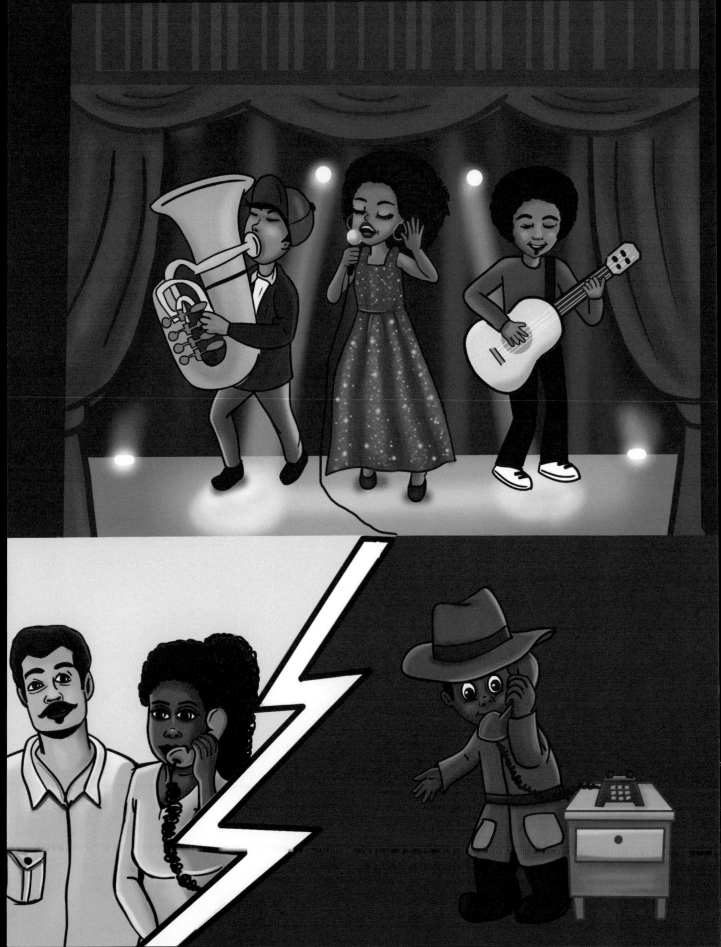

In my dreams, I am a private detective spy;
here to be these parents' extra eyes.
Scurrying around, looking for clues …
I discover their daughter's been studying
and secretly singing jazz blues.
She's part of a band with Brad and Louis,
making amazing music.
Surely this will be good news or maybe their daughter
has some explaining to do!

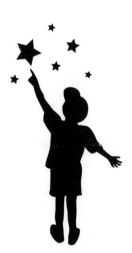

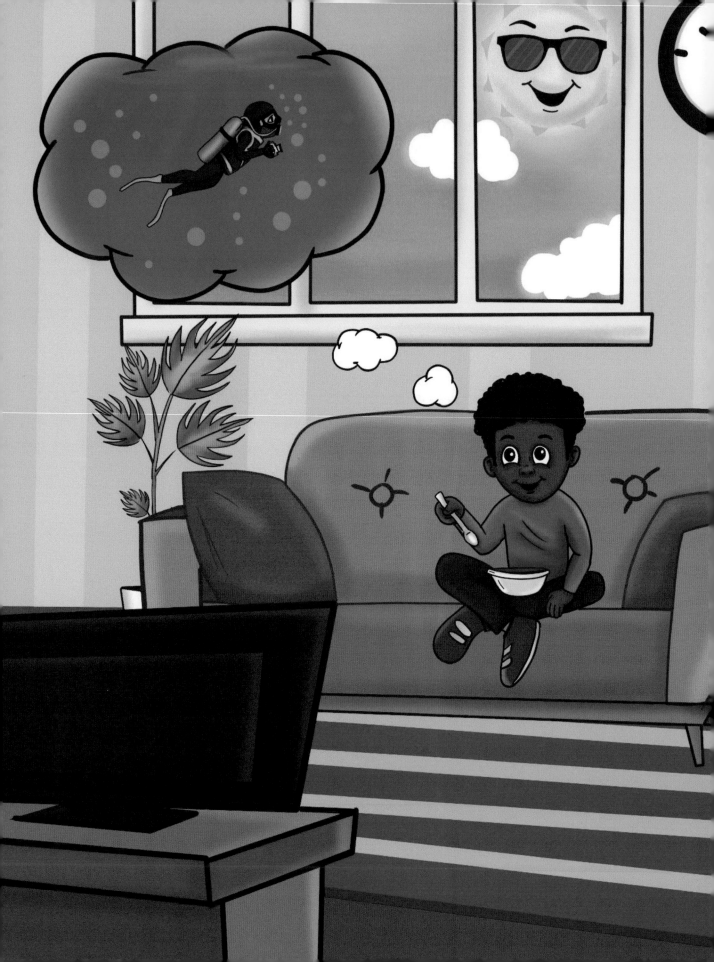

Up in the morning, the sun is high;
wish I could go for a deep-sea dive.
Back to the telly, as I watch cartoons and eat jelly.
I can't wait for bed!

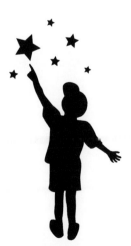

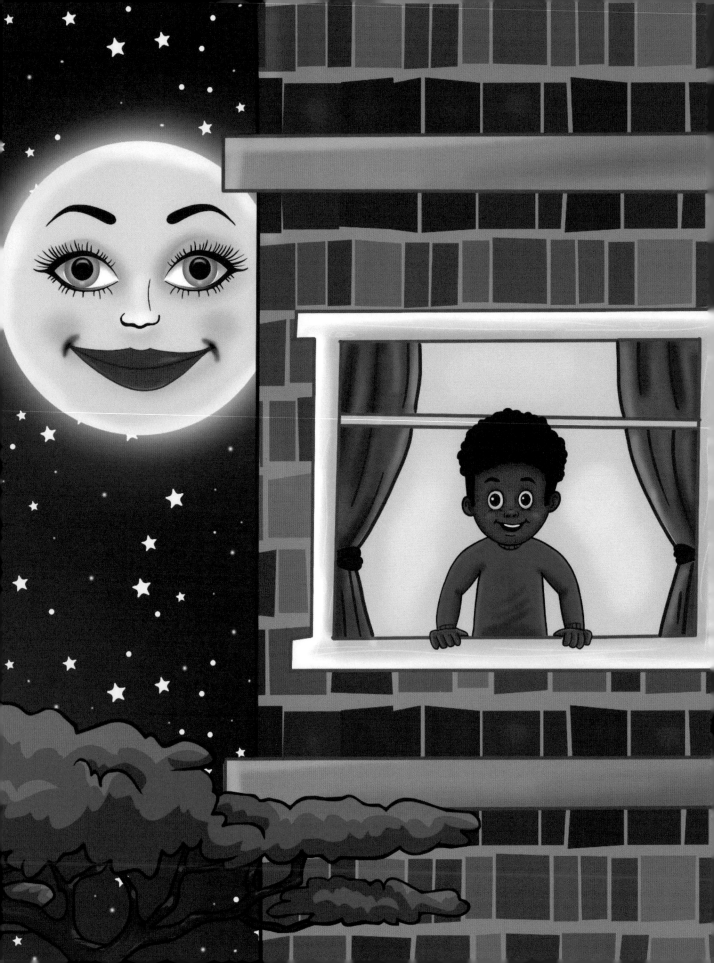

As I count the stars at night, my mother comes in
and says "sleep tight".
She tucks me in and kisses my chin.
This is where my journey begins!

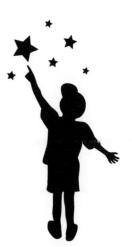

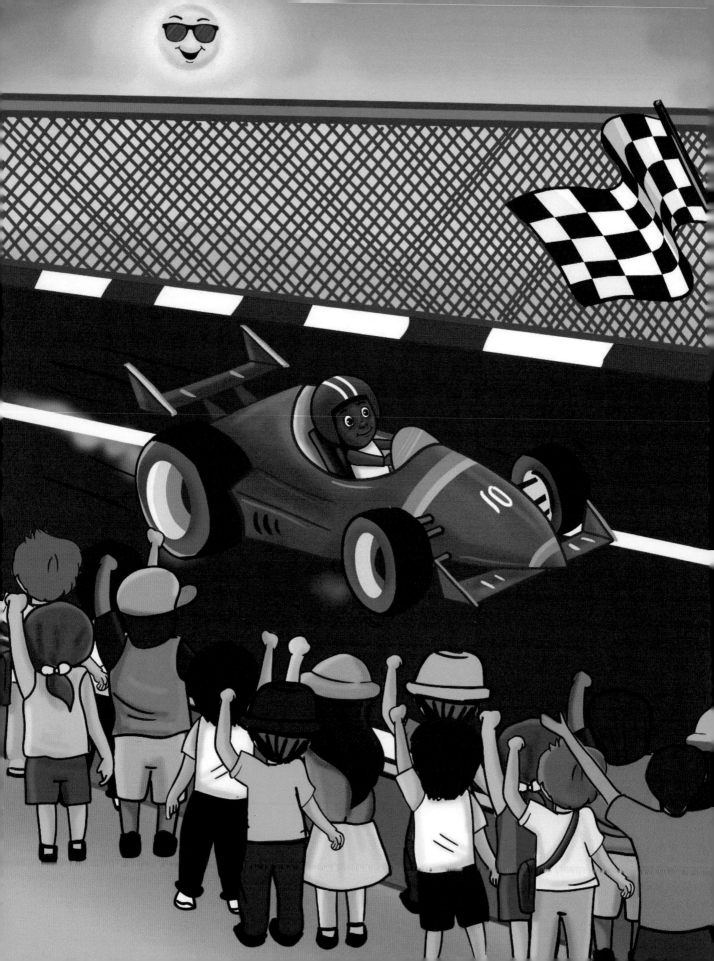

In my dreams I am a Formula One racer,
showing off skills in my speedy red car.
A ZOOOOOM and a BOOOOM as I approach the bend,
gripping the wheel tight, steady on the brakes.
The crowd cheers as I recover from fright.
Excitement fulfils me, as I approach the chequered flag.
Coming first, I might add!

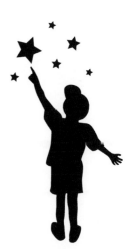

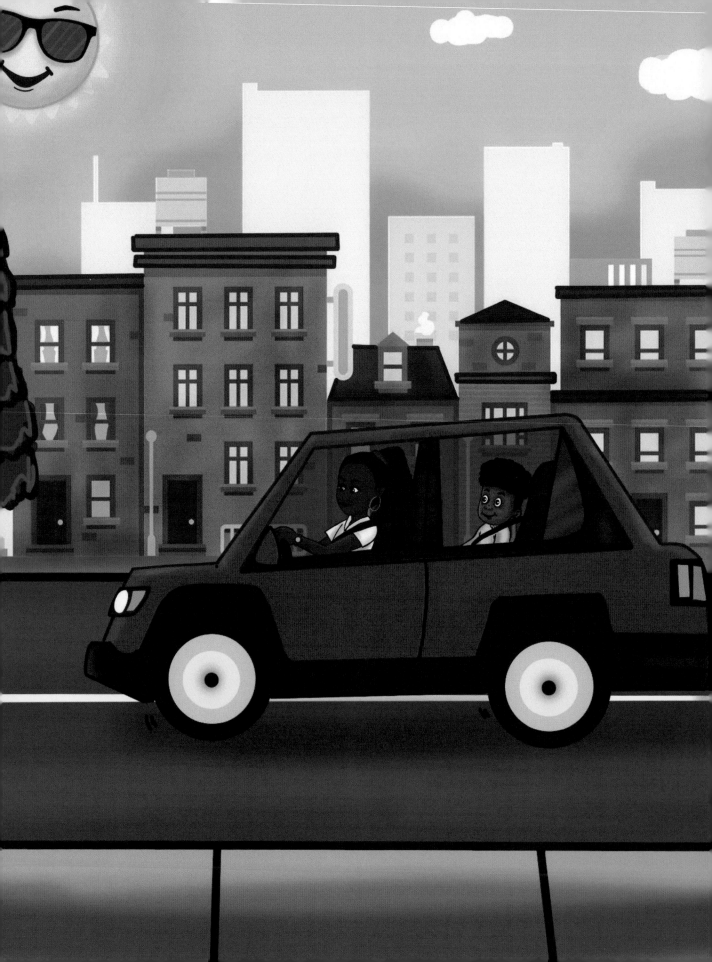

I am up early, with not much to do,
going to the shops with my mum, to avoid the morning moods.
I daydream about vivid, colourful adventures,
swirling around in my head.
I can't wait for bed!

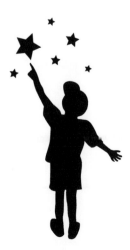

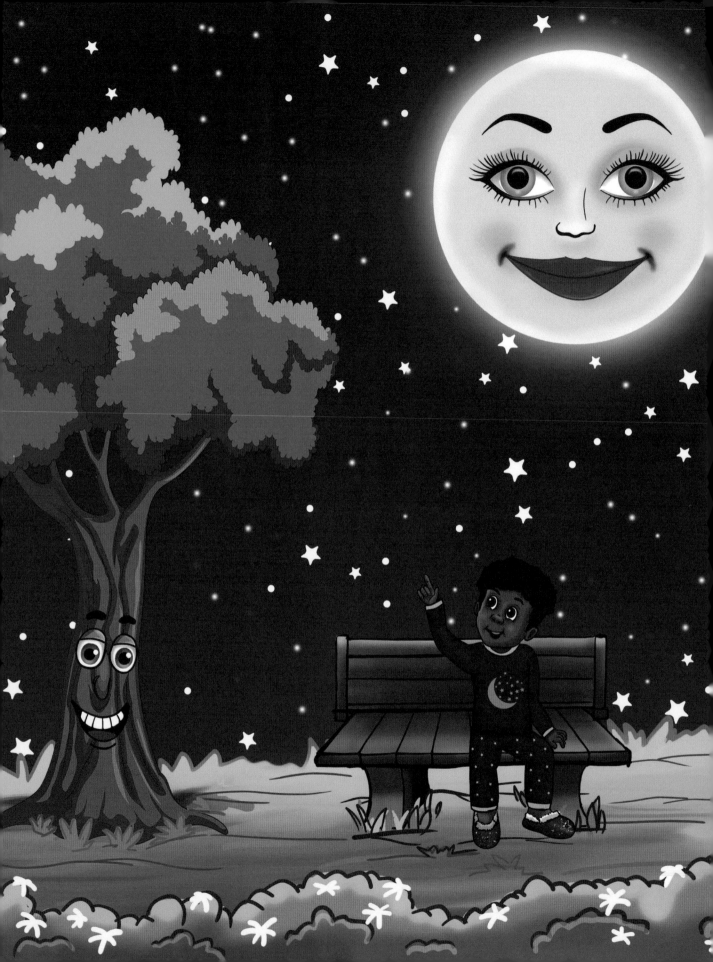

As I count the stars at night, my mother comes in
and says "sleep tight".
She tucks me in and kisses my chin.
This is where my journey begins!

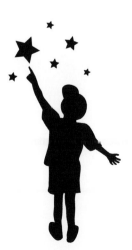

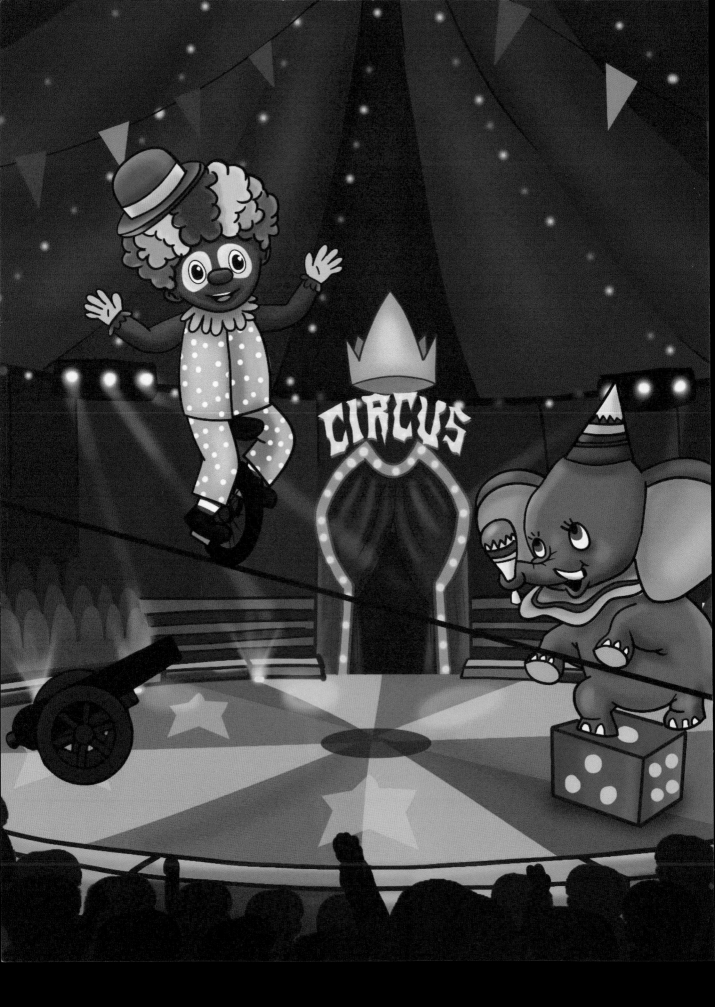

In my dreams, I am a circus clown, here to amaze the town,
balancing on a tightrope whilst making funny jokes.
Riding a one-wheeled bike with an elephant bravely balancing
on a dice – she's boldly holding on for dear life.
I take a much-deserved bow, I hear the whispers of all the possibilities
and how the crowd's so stunned all they can say is WOW!
"Encore, encore, we want more;
can you shoot from the rocket over there on the floor?"
"What an amazing show," they scream,
"you and elephant make a great team!"

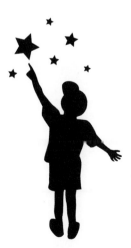

16

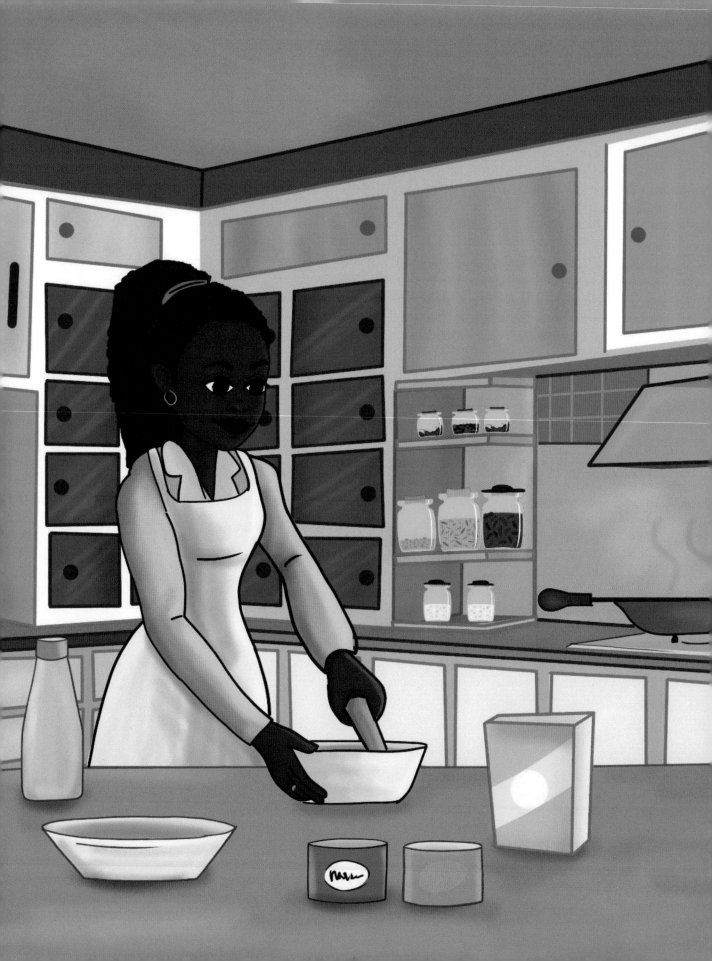

I'm up in the morning, still yawning.

What an amazing night; the dreams were vibrant and bright.

Mother's making cookies, to cheer me up, I guess.

I wish I could do all those amazing things and really go on

these magical adventures with all the sights to be seen.

Stories, adventures bubbling in my head!

I can't wait for bed.

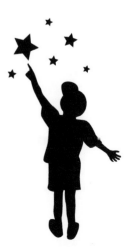

18

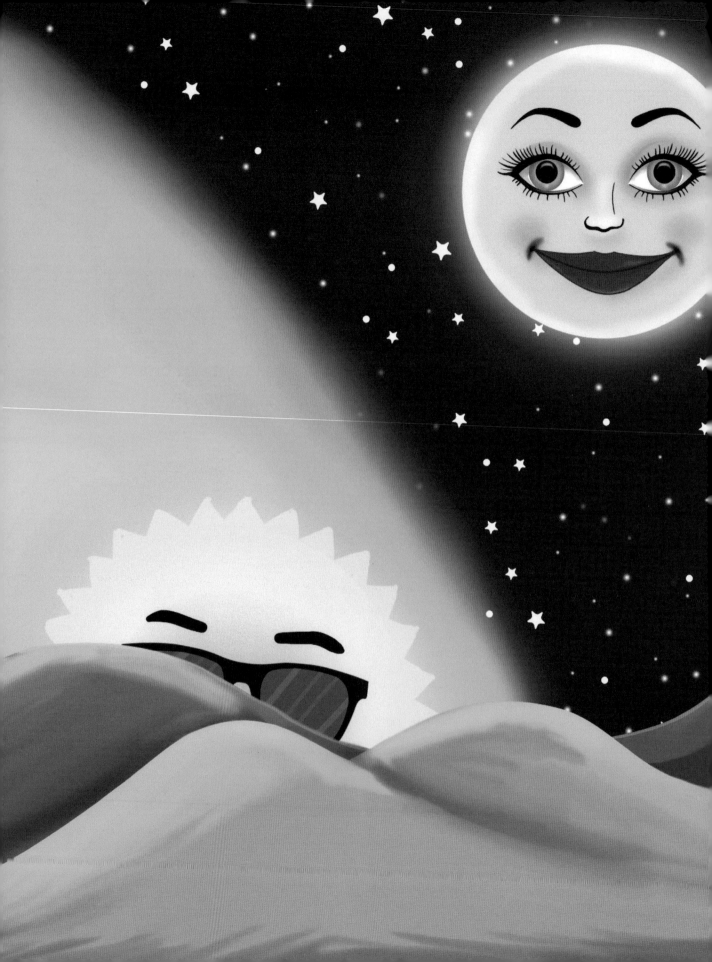

As I count the stars at night, my mother comes in
and says "sleep tight".
She tucks me in and kisses my chin.
This is where my journey begins!

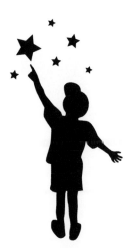

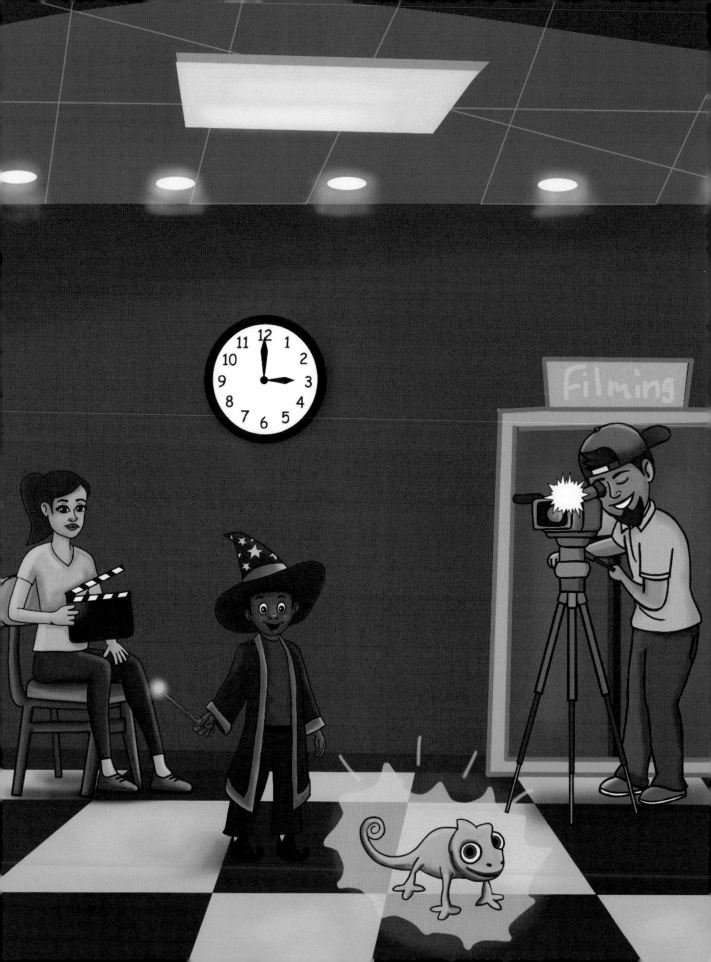

In my dreams I am a famous star,

performing action movies for the cinema.

From being on the big screen, to winning awards

and even meeting the Queen!

I win the part to act as a wizard that turns the villain into a slimy lizard.

Then I walk through a hurricane blizzard to save the Good Witch

of the West, putting my magic to the ultimate test.

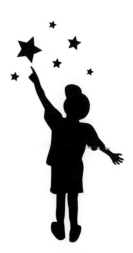

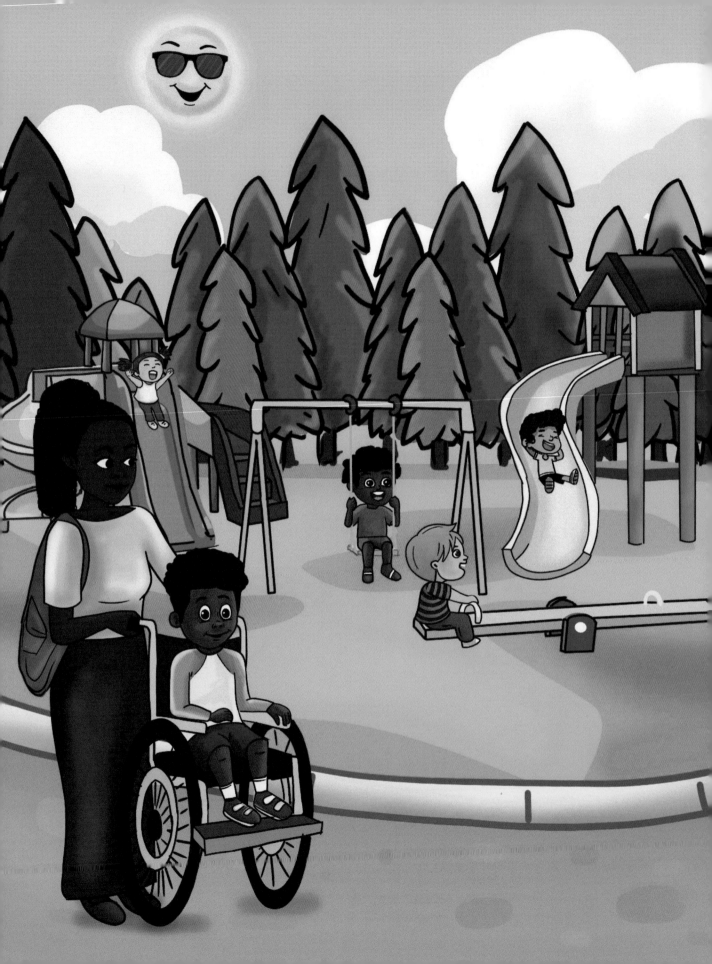

I am up early in the morning; it's a bright sunny day.

I am off to the park, where I can go have fun and play.

Mum pushes my wheelchair over to the swings,

feeling the wonderful warm air on my skin.

I wish I had friends who were kind and friendly.

We would play fun games and learn we are all really just the same

and the only real difference is our names.

I can't wait for bed!

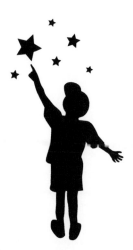

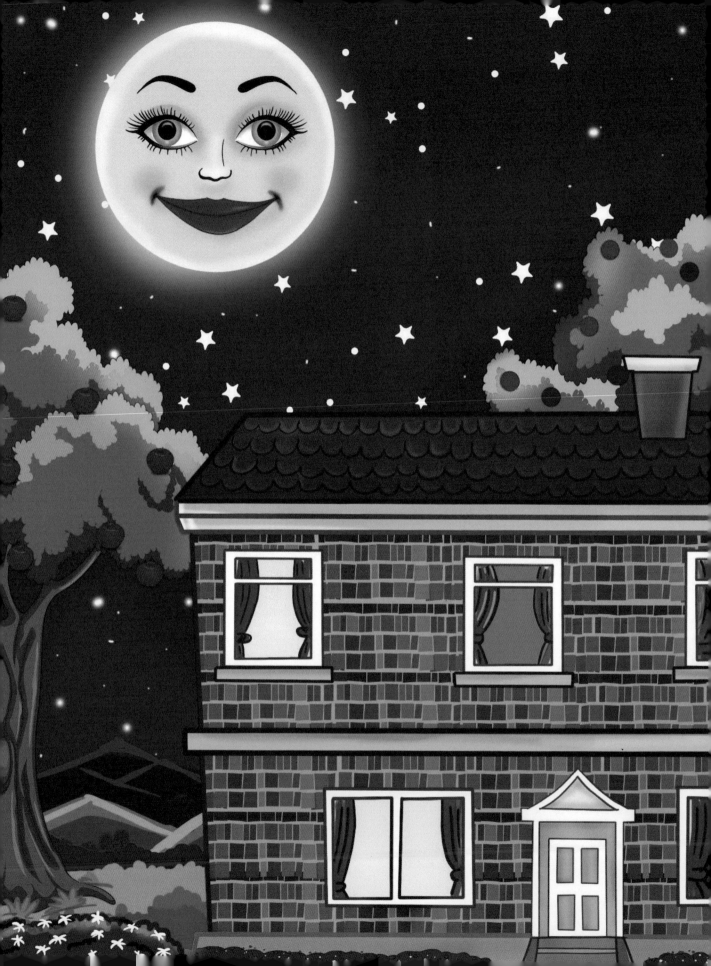

As I count the stars at night, my mother comes in
and says "sleep tight".
She tucks me in and kisses my chin.
This is where my journey begins!

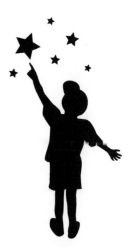

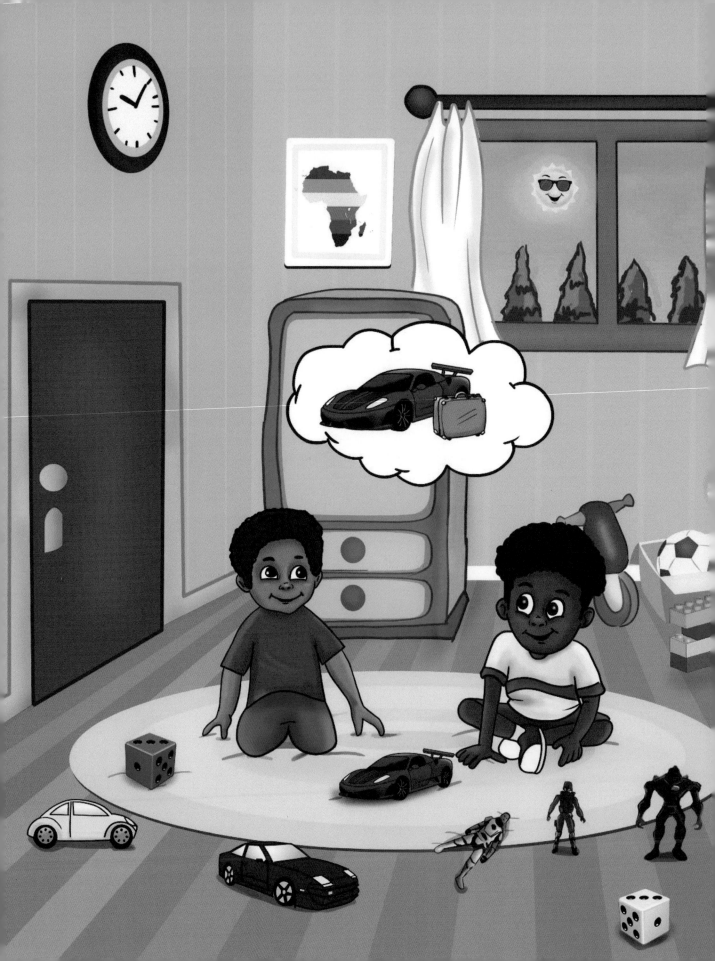

In my dreams, I play with my new friend.

I wish this imaginary play would never end.

We dress up and pretend to be businessmen,

driving around in our fancy flash cars.

We have happy faces, holding our business briefcases,

whisked around the world in a day.

Living lavish – what more can one say?

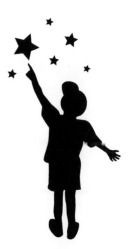

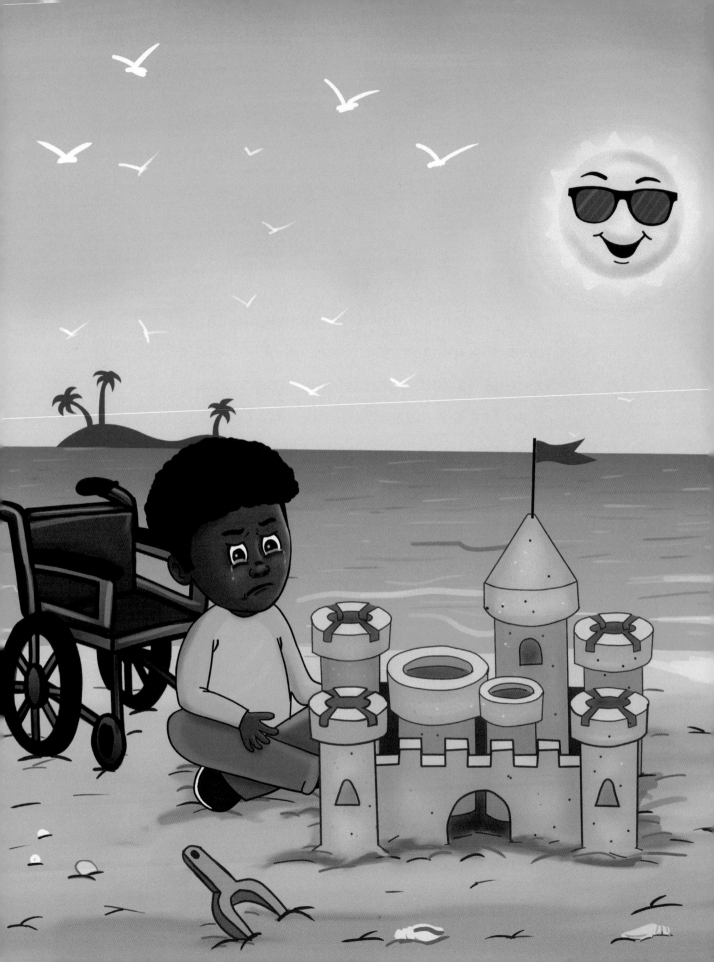

I am up early in the morning, on this fine sunny day.
I am off to the seaside where I can sit and play.
Maybe I'll build sandcastles and eat ice-cream all day.

"That sounds like fun, Yayyyy!"

Seeing the birds drift off into the sky, I look up and begin to sigh,
as a heavy tear rolls out of my eye.
In my dreams, I'm an exciting human being. When I am awake,
playing alone makes my thoughts race to the ceiling.
I want to share my deepest secrets: like I am really scared of
the mornings, because they can be so dull and boring.

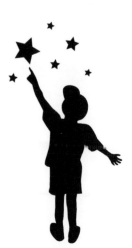

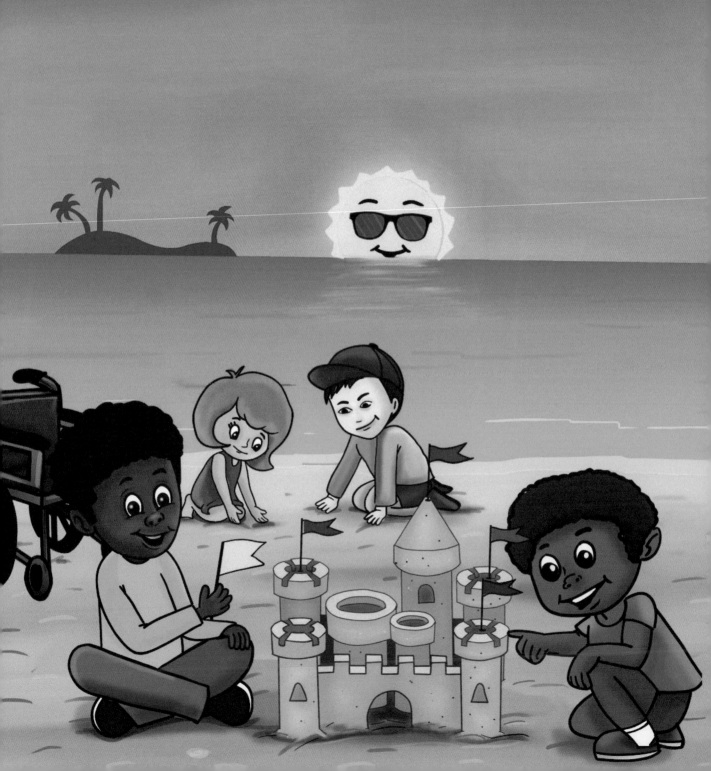

The last flag goes up on my sandcastle;

taking a moment to sit and be still.

Children playing all around; all you can hear is cheerful sounds.

I am no longer alone. A boy comes over and says,

"Hi, my name is Ben and I'd like to be your friend.

Maybe we could pretend that your sandcastle has sea monsters

and we could be the town's heroes."

Other children see the fun and come closer until they are sitting

with us in the lovely hot sun, asking lots of question

about the hard work we have done.

The sun is long gone – but the fun and games have just begun.

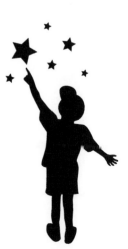

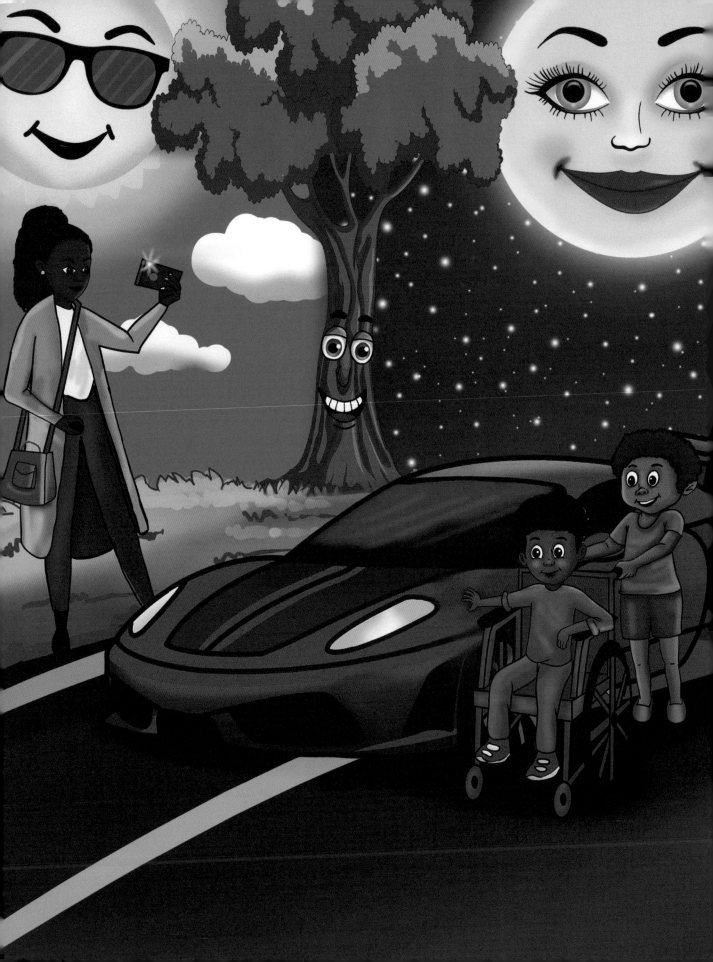

I had an amazing day.

I made a friend and plans are already made.

We will meet again someday soon;

I can't wait to show him the toys in my room.

I finally see that I can be me and not only in my dreams,

but in real life I am an amazing human being, who deserves

friendships that are caring, filled with laughter and sharing.

Just like me, you can use your imagination

and create a world of fascination.

During the day, I used to mope around, lonely and sad.

All I needed was courage in my heart

and it came from within from the start.

Now I believe that not only in my dreams am I capable

of doing the most surprising things.

Get ready to begin exploring, and finally, just like that ...

We can begin to love our mornings.

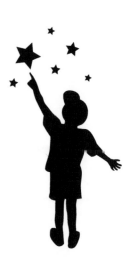

Write your dreams here:

_____

_____

_____

_____

_____

_____

_____

_____

_____

_____

_____

_____

Write your dreams here:

About The Author

Michelle Marshall was born in the wintry months of December 1983 in London, UK. From a young age Michelle was drawn to writing and contributed at every opportunity in school to write poems and storybooks, which engaged children and teachers, who were captivated by her vivid and colourful imagination. Michelle uses creativity as a form of expression in her writing.

Upcoming into the writing scene Michelle has high aspirations and visions to write children's books, poetry and other creative outlets for both adults and children. Her books will be drawn from her life experiences as a form of inspirational perspective to encourage, motivate and build positive images of the world we live in.

Michelle wrote In My Dreams to inspire everyone who reads this book to create positive thinking patterns and belief systems. This book is to inspire children to create a positive mental attitude from a young age.

Michelle strongly believes that mental health, disability and race, due to their sensitive nature, are amongst the many topics not discussed frequently within the education system and society.

Having this in mind, Michelle wants to help children and families build stronger bonds through reading time with her books that assist readers to be inspired and build connections.

"If we are to create a society of acceptance we must first create understanding and then we will have unity."

Writing is Michelle's passion, and she has a powerful insight she would love to share with the world to motivate those who have limiting beliefs of any kind and, more importantly, to encourage them to believe in themselves and all the possibilities life has to offer.

Website:

   www.michellemarshall.co.uk

   Michelle Marshall

   Inmydreams2022

Printed in Great Britain
by Amazon